GERIATRIC POCKET GUIDE
LONG TERM CARE EDITION

DR. MOHAMED ELGENDY
LMCC, CCFP, CANADA

DISCLAIMER

This pocket guide was developed with the assistance of advanced AI tools to streamline content generation. Every chapter has been thoroughly reviewed, edited, and authenticated by Dr. Mohamed Elgendy, LMCC, CCFP (Canada), ensuring accuracy, credibility, and clinical authenticity. The result is a modern, innovative reference that blends the efficiency of AI with the rigor of professional medical expertise

This pocket guide summarizes common geriatric and long-term care approaches using only open-access guidance; no proprietary or subscription-based content is reproduced.

Clinical descriptions (including assessments, investigations, and treatments) are abbreviated for educational purposes and exam preparation. They are not intended as complete protocols or substitutes for independent clinical judgment.

Management should always be performed within the clinician's scope of training, local regulations, and available resources, with appropriate patient consent, monitoring, and safety measures. Escalate care promptly when red flags arise (e.g., acute delirium, sudden functional decline, new or worsening confusion, falls with suspected fracture, sepsis, uncontrolled pain, medication toxicity, or complex multi-morbidity) or when the situation exceeds your competence or resources.

Always confirm current local and national guidelines, product monographs/labels, and institutional pathways before application. Verify patient-specific contraindications, comorbidities, goals of care, advance directives, and drug interactions. Clinical responsibility remains with the treating clinician.

ABOUT THE AUTHOR

Dr. Mohamed Elgendy is a licensed Canadian physician with the Licentiate of the Medical Council of Canada (LMCC) and Certification in Family Medicine (CCFP) from the College of Family Physicians of Canada.

He has extensive hands-on experience as both a rural emergency physician and family doctor, currently practicing in Saskatchewan, Canada. With a deep commitment to improving emergency and acute care in underserved communities, Dr. Elgendy focuses on practical, evidence-based emergency medicine adapted to the realities of rural practice.

His work bridges the gap between academic guidelines and frontline clinical realities, offering accessible, concise resources to help clinicians make confident, lifesaving decisions in resource-limited settings.

DEDICATION

This guide is dedicated to the patients in rural and remote communities—whose resilience and courage inspire every clinical decision; to the clinicians, nurses, medics, and allied staff who deliver essential emergency care with skill and compassion despite distance, resource limitations, and isolation; to mentors and colleagues who freely share knowledge so that care remains safe and evidence-informed; and to my family, whose unwavering support sustains this work.

May this concise, open-access emergency pocket guide serve them all.

— Dr. Mohamed Elgendy

TABLE OF CONTENTS

v

1. GENERAL CARE IN LTC

CHAPTER 1
Comprehensive Geriatric Assessment (CGA)

Overview

CGA is a multidimensional diagnostic process to assess the medical, psychological, and functional capabilities of older adults. In LTC, it supports individualized care planning and improves outcomes by integrating medical, functional, cognitive, and social domains.

Risk Factors / Epidemiology

- Advanced age, frailty, multimorbidity
- Polypharmacy, cognitive impairment
- Functional decline, recurrent hospitalizations
- Social isolation, caregiver burden

Clinical Presentation

- Decline in mobility, ADLs, or cognition
- Frequent falls, delirium, malnutrition
- Multiple chronic conditions

Assessment / Investigations

- Medical: comorbidities, medications
- Functional: ADLs, mobility, continence
- Cognitive: MMSE, MoCA
- Social: support systems, living situation
- Nutritional: weight, BMI, labs
- Mental health: depression, anxiety screening

Management

Non-pharmacological:

- Multidisciplinary team approach
- Individualized care plans
- Rehabilitation and social engagement
- Advanced care planning discussions

Pharmacological:

- Medication review for polypharmacy
- Optimize chronic disease management
- Avoid high-risk medications

References (Open-Access)

- NHS – Comprehensive geriatric assessment: https://www.nhs.uk/conditions/geriatrician/
- Public Health Agency of Canada – Seniors care: https://www.canada.ca/en/public-health

CHAPTER 2
Activities of Daily Living (ADLs) and Independence Support

Overview

ADLs are basic self-care tasks including bathing, dressing, feeding, toileting, and mobility. Maintaining independence in ADLs is a major goal in LTC, as it enhances dignity and quality of life.

Risk Factors / Epidemiology

- Frailty, dementia, Parkinson's, stroke
- Depression, social isolation
- Sensory impairments
- Environmental hazards

Clinical Presentation

- Dependence in bathing, dressing, toileting, feeding
- Loss of mobility, transfers
- Decline in instrumental ADLs (shopping, cooking, finances)

Assessment / Investigations

- Katz Index of Independence in ADLs
- Barthel Index
- Occupational therapy assessment
- Review of living environment and safety

Management

Non-pharmacological:

- Assistive devices, environmental modifications
- Physiotherapy, occupational therapy
- Encourage participation in ADLs with supervision
- Promote group and recreational activities

Pharmacological:

- No direct drug therapy; manage underlying medical contributors (pain, depression, Parkinson's)

References (Open-Access)

- NHS – Activities of daily living:
  https://www.nhs.uk/conditions/social-care-and-support-guide/practical-tips-if-you-care-for-someone/
- Public Health Agency of Canada – Healthy aging:
  https://www.canada.ca/en/public-health/services/health-promotion/aging-seniors.html

CHAPTER 3
Polypharmacy and Deprescribing

Overview

Polypharmacy (use of ≥5 medications) is common in LTC and increases the risk of adverse drug events, falls, delirium, and hospitalizations. Deprescribing is the planned process of dose reduction or stopping medications that may no longer be beneficial or may be harmful.

Risk Factors / Epidemiology

- Advanced age, multimorbidity
- Multiple prescribers, poor documentation
- Lack of regular medication reviews
- Cognitive impairment, poor adherence

Clinical Presentation

- Falls, delirium, functional decline
- Adverse drug reactions (bleeding, hypoglycemia)
- Polypharmacy burden (pill load, cost)

Assessment / Investigations

- Regular medication reconciliation
- Tools: Beers Criteria, STOPP/START criteria
- Evaluate drug–drug and drug–disease interactions
- Assess goals of care and prognosis

Management

Non-pharmacological:

- Education of staff and families
- Shared decision-making on deprescribing
- Monitor withdrawal symptoms and recurrence of illness

Pharmacological:

- Prioritize deprescribing sedatives, anticholinergics, PPIs, and duplicate therapies
- Taper benzodiazepines gradually (e.g., lorazepam reduce by 25% every 2–3 weeks)
- Replace with safer alternatives when appropriate (e.g., SSRIs for anxiety, non-drug sleep strategies)

References (Open-Access)

- Canadian Deprescribing Network: https://deprescribing.org
- NHS – Medicines and side effects: https://www.nhs.uk/medicines/

CHAPTER 4
Advance Care Planning & Goals of Care

Overview

Advance Care Planning (ACP) is a process that supports adults in understanding and sharing their personal values, goals, and preferences for future medical care. In LTC, ACP ensures that residents receive care aligned with their wishes and reduces unnecessary hospital transfers.

Risk Factors / Epidemiology

- Advanced age, multimorbidity, dementia
- Frequent hospitalizations
- Lack of family or substitute decision maker
- Cultural and language barriers

Clinical Presentation

- Discussions initiated during admission or decline
- Expression of care preferences (comfort vs. curative)
- Formal documents: advance directives, POLST/MOST forms

Assessment / Investigations

- Review existing directives and legal documents
- Assess decision-making capacity
- Involve family and substitute decision makers

Management

Non-pharmacological:

- Structured ACP discussions by trained staff
- Documentation of resident wishes in care plan
- Regular review as conditions change
- Use interpreters and culturally sensitive approaches

Pharmacological:

- Not applicable, but relevant to medication decisions (e.g., stopping statins in palliative phase)

References (Open-Access)

- Canadian Hospice Palliative Care Association – Advance Care Planning:
  https://www.advancecareplanning.ca
- NHS – Planning your care:
  https://www.nhs.uk/conditions/end-of-life-care/planning-ahead/

CHAPTER 5
Palliative and End-of-Life Care

Overview

Palliative care in LTC focuses on quality of life, symptom management, and support for residents and families at the end of life. It emphasizes comfort, dignity, and minimizing unnecessary interventions.

Risk Factors / Epidemiology

- Advanced age, multimorbidity, terminal illness
- Dementia, advanced frailty
- Frequent hospitalizations or functional decline

Clinical Presentation

- Pain, dyspnea, delirium, fatigue, anorexia
- Declining function, weight loss
- Family distress and caregiver burden

Assessment / Investigations

- Symptom assessment tools (e.g., ESAS)
- Prognostic indicators (Palliative Performance Scale)
- Review medication appropriateness

Management

Non-pharmacological:

- Emotional, spiritual, psychosocial support
- Interdisciplinary team care
- Family meetings, counseling, bereavement support

Pharmacological:

- Pain: Morphine 2.5 mg PO q4h PRN; Hydromorphone 0.25–0.5 mg q4–6h PRN
- Dyspnea: Opioids as above; oxygen if hypoxemic
- Delirium: Haloperidol 0.25–0.5 mg PO/SC BID–TID
- Nausea: Metoclopramide 5–10 mg PO/SC TID
- Constipation prevention: Senna 8.6 mg PO HS ± Lactulose 15 mL daily

References (Open-Access)

- Canadian Hospice Palliative Care Association: https://www.chpca.ca
- NHS – End of life care: https://www.nhs.uk/conditions/end-of-life-care/

CHAPTER 6
Ethical and Legal Considerations

Overview

Ethical and legal issues in LTC include consent, capacity, substitute decision-making, confidentiality, and equitable access to care. Staff must balance autonomy, beneficence, and safety while adhering to laws and ethical codes.

Risk Factors / Epidemiology

- Cognitive impairment, dementia
- Limited decision-making capacity
- Cultural and language barriers
- Variable family involvement

Clinical Presentation

- Ethical dilemmas in life-sustaining treatment
- Conflicts between families and staff
- Unclear legal documents or advance directives

Assessment / Investigations

- Capacity assessments
- Review of consent forms and directives
- Legal consultation when needed

Management

Non-pharmacological:

- Ethics consultation and team discussion
- Transparent communication with families
- Documentation of decisions and rationale

- Staff training in ethics and legal issues

Pharmacological:

- Not directly applicable; relates to care planning and consent for interventions

References (Open-Access)

- Government of Canada – Consent and capacity:
  https://www.canada.ca/en/public-health
- NHS – End of life decisions and ethics:
  https://www.nhs.uk/conditions/end-of-life-care/

2. MEDICAL CONDITIONS COMMON IN LTC – NEUROLOGY / PSYCHIATRY

CHAPTER 7
Dementia (Alzheimer's, Vascular, Lewy Body)

Overview

Dementia is a progressive decline in cognitive function affecting memory, reasoning, and daily activities. Alzheimer's disease is the most common type, followed by vascular dementia and Lewy body dementia. Management in LTC focuses on safety, behavioral symptoms, and caregiver support.

Risk Factors / Epidemiology

- Advanced age
- Family history, genetics (APOE4)
- Vascular risk factors (HTN, diabetes, smoking)
- Parkinson's disease and synucleinopathies (Lewy body dementia)

Clinical Presentation

- Memory loss, disorientation, language impairment
- Personality/behavior changes, hallucinations (Lewy body)
- Executive dysfunction (vascular dementia)
- Functional decline, wandering, incontinence in later stages

Assessment / Investigations

- Cognitive testing: MMSE, MoCA
- Depression screening (rule out pseudodementia)
- Labs: CBC, electrolytes, TSH, B12, glucose

- Imaging: CT/MRI to rule out structural lesions, vascular disease

Management

Non-pharmacological:

- Structured routines, orientation cues
- Safe wandering areas, environmental modifications
- Recreational and cognitive stimulation programs
- Staff and caregiver education

Pharmacological:

- Alzheimer's: Donepezil 5 mg PO daily (increase to 10 mg after 4–6 weeks); Rivastigmine 1.5 mg PO BID → 6 mg BID; Memantine 5 mg daily → 10 mg BID
- Vascular dementia: Optimize BP, diabetes, lipid control; antiplatelets if prior stroke/TIA
- Lewy body: Avoid antipsychotics if possible; if needed, quetiapine 12.5–25 mg HS cautiously
- Treat depression/anxiety with SSRIs (Sertraline 25–50 mg daily)

References (Open-Access)

- Alzheimer Society of Canada: https://alzheimer.ca
- NHS – Dementia overview: https://www.nhs.uk/conditions/dementia/

CHAPTER 8
Delirium Recognition & Prevention

Overview

Delirium is an acute, fluctuating disturbance in attention and cognition. It is common in LTC residents, often triggered by infection, medications, or metabolic disturbances. It is associated with high morbidity and mortality.

Risk Factors / Epidemiology

- Advanced age, dementia, sensory impairment
- Polypharmacy, recent hospitalization
- Infection, dehydration, electrolyte imbalance

Clinical Presentation

- Acute onset, fluctuating course
- Inattention, disorganized thinking
- Altered level of consciousness
- Hyperactive (agitation) or hypoactive (lethargy) forms

Assessment / Investigations

- CAM (Confusion Assessment Method)
- Labs: CBC, electrolytes, renal/liver function, glucose, urinalysis
- Imaging or LP if CNS infection suspected
- Review medications (anticholinergics, opioids, sedatives)

Management

Non-pharmacological:

- Identify and treat underlying cause (infection, dehydration, medications)
- Orientation cues, clocks, calendars
- Mobilization, hydration, vision/hearing aids
- Quiet environment, sleep hygiene

Pharmacological:

- Avoid sedatives/anticholinergics if possible
- Severe agitation jeopardizing safety: Haloperidol 0.25–0.5 mg PO/SC q8h (use lowest effective dose)
- Avoid benzodiazepines unless alcohol/benzo withdrawal suspected

References (Open-Access)

- NHS–Delirium: https://www.nhs.uk/conditions/confusion/
- Public Health Agency of Canada – Seniors' mental health: https://www.canada.ca/en/public-health

CHAPTER 9
Parkinson's Disease

Overview

Parkinson's disease (PD) is a progressive neurodegenerative disorder characterized by motor and non-motor symptoms. Management in LTC emphasizes motor symptom control, fall prevention, and non-motor care.

Risk Factors / Epidemiology

- Advanced age
- Family history, environmental exposures
- Male sex
- Lewy body pathology

Clinical Presentation

- Bradykinesia, resting tremor, rigidity, postural instability
- Hypophonia, dysphagia, drooling
- Depression, cognitive decline, hallucinations

Assessment / Investigations

- Clinical diagnosis; response to levodopa supports diagnosis
- Rule out drug-induced parkinsonism (antipsychotics, metoclopramide)
- Cognitive screening for dementia in PD

Management

Non-pharmacological:

- Physiotherapy, occupational therapy
- Speech therapy for hypophonia/dysphagia
- Fall prevention, mobility aids
- Nutrition and constipation management

Pharmacological:

- Levodopa/carbidopa: 100/25 mg PO TID; titrate to effect (monitor dyskinesias, orthostasis)
- Dopamine agonists (pramipexole, ropinirole) generally avoided in elderly (confusion, hallucinations)
- MAO-B inhibitors (rasagiline, selegiline) rarely used in frail elderly
- Manage hallucinations with quetiapine 12.5–25 mg PO HS if needed

References (Open-Access)

- Parkinson Canada: https://www.parkinson.ca
- NHS – Parkinson's disease: https://www.nhs.uk/conditions/parkinsons-disease/

CHAPTER 10
Stroke Recovery in LTC

Overview

Stroke is a leading cause of disability in LTC residents. Management focuses on secondary prevention, rehabilitation, and maximizing independence.

Risk Factors / Epidemiology

- Hypertension, diabetes, atrial fibrillation
- Prior stroke or TIA
- Advanced age, smoking, hyperlipidemia

Clinical Presentation

- Residual hemiparesis, dysphagia, aphasia
- Cognitive impairment, depression
- Risk of recurrent stroke, aspiration pneumonia

Assessment / Investigations

- Neurological exam, mobility and ADL assessment
- Swallowing assessment for aspiration risk
- Monitor BP, glucose, lipids

Management

Non-pharmacological:

- Physiotherapy, occupational therapy, speech therapy
- Assistive devices for mobility and communication
- Dysphagia management (texture-modified diets)
- Social and psychological support]

Pharmacological:

- Antiplatelet therapy: ASA 81 mg PO daily or Clopidogrel 75 mg PO daily
- Anticoagulation if atrial fibrillation present (see AF management)
- Statins (e.g., Atorvastatin 20–40 mg PO daily)
- Control of BP, diabetes, lipids as per guidelines

References (Open-Access)

- Heart & Stroke Foundation of Canada – Stroke: https://www.heartandstroke.ca
- NHS – Stroke rehabilitation: https://www.nhs.uk/conditions/stroke/recovery/

CHAPTER 11
Depression and Anxiety in Elderly

Overview

Depression and anxiety are common but underdiagnosed in LTC. They worsen outcomes by increasing disability, mortality, and caregiver burden. Management includes psychosocial interventions and cautious use of medications.

Risk Factors / Epidemiology

- Social isolation, bereavement
- Dementia, chronic pain, disability
- Polypharmacy, medical comorbidities
- History of mood or anxiety disorders

Clinical Presentation

- Persistent sadness, anhedonia
- Anxiety, irritability, restlessness
- Sleep disturbance, appetite change
- Somatic complaints, functional decline

Assessment / Investigations

- Geriatric Depression Scale (GDS)
- PHQ-9, GAD-7 if feasible
- Rule out delirium, hypothyroidism, B12 deficiency

Management

Non-pharmacological:

- Supportive counseling, CBT, group therapy
- Physical activity, social engagement

- Address sleep hygiene, pain control

Pharmacological:

- SSRIs: Sertraline 25–50 mg PO daily; Citalopram 10–20 mg PO daily (max 20 mg in elderly)
- SNRIs: Duloxetine 30 mg PO daily (also for neuropathic pain)
- Mirtazapine 7.5–15 mg PO HS (for depression + insomnia)
- Avoid TCAs and benzodiazepines due to side effects

References (Open-Access)

- NHS – Depression in older adults:
  https://www.nhs.uk/mental-health/conditions/depression/older-people/
- Public Health Agency of Canada – Mental health and seniors:
  https://www.canada.ca/en/public-health

CHAPTER 12
Sleep Disorders

Overview

Sleep disorders in LTC include insomnia, sleep apnea, restless legs syndrome, and REM sleep behavior disorder. They contribute to falls, delirium, and functional decline. Non-pharmacological measures are first-line.

Risk Factors / Epidemiology

- Advanced age, frailty
- Dementia, depression, Parkinson's, stroke
- Polypharmacy (sedatives, anticholinergics)
- Pain, nocturia, chronic illness

Clinical Presentation

- Difficulty initiating/maintaining sleep
- Daytime fatigue, irritability, confusion
- Snoring, witnessed apneas
- Nocturnal behaviors (dream enactment in RBD)

Assessment / Investigations

- Sleep history, diaries if feasible
- STOP-Bang questionnaire for OSA
- Labs: TSH, ferritin if RLS suspected
- Medication review for sedating/deliriogenic drugs

Management

Non-pharmacological:

- Sleep hygiene: regular bedtime/wake time, avoid caffeine/alcohol, reduce nighttime noise
- Bright light exposure, daytime activity
- Treat underlying contributors (pain, nocturia)

Pharmacological:

- Insomnia: Melatonin 1–3 mg PO HS; Doxepin 3–6 mg HS; Mirtazapine 7.5–15 mg HS if depression coexists
- RLS: Iron supplementation if ferritin <75 µg/L; Gabapentin 100–300 mg HS (renal adjust)
- RBD: Melatonin 3–6 mg HS; Clonazepam 0.25–0.5 mg HS with caution
- Avoid benzodiazepines and Z-drugs when possible

References (Open-Access)

- NHS – Insomnia:
  https://www.nhs.uk/conditions/insomnia/
- Canadian Deprescribing Network – Benzodiazepine resources: https://deprescribing.org
- National Institute on Aging – Sleep and aging: https://www.nia.nih.gov

B.) MEDICAL CONDITIONS COMMON IN LTC – CARDIOVASCULAR

CHAPTER 13
Hypertension in Frail Elderly

Overview

Hypertension is highly prevalent in frail LTC residents. Management prioritizes reduction of stroke, heart failure, and symptomatic hypotension, while minimizing polypharmacy and adverse effects. Targets are individualized; moderate control is often appropriate in frailty.

Risk Factors / Epidemiology

- Advanced age, arterial stiffness, atherosclerosis
- Diabetes, CKD, sleep apnea
- Polypharmacy (NSAIDs, steroids, SNRIs may raise BP)
- Autonomic dysfunction and orthostatic hypotension risk

Clinical Presentation

- Often asymptomatic; may present with headaches, dizziness
- Orthostatic symptoms (lightheadedness, falls) with overtreatment
- End-organ disease: LVH, CKD, cerebrovascular disease

Assessment / Investigations

- Measure seated and standing BP (orthostatic change ≥20 systolic or ≥10 diastolic is significant)
- Review medications and sodium intake; assess adherence
- Labs: electrolytes, creatinine/eGFR, ACR (albumin/creatinine ratio), lipids; ECG for LVH/AF

Management

Non-pharmacological:

- Individualize BP targets (commonly SBP 130–150 mmHg in frail elderly; avoid SBP <120 if symptomatic)
- Reduce sodium intake, encourage gentle physical activity, weight optimization, limit alcohol
- Manage sleep apnea and pain; review and deprescribe BP-raising drugs

Pharmacological (start low, go slow; check orthostatics and renal function):

- Thiazide(-like) diuretics: Hydrochlorothiazide 12.5 mg PO daily (up to 25 mg); Indapamide 1.25 mg PO daily
- ACE inhibitors: Perindopril 2–4 mg PO daily (titrate); Lisinopril 5 mg PO daily (2.5–40 mg range)
- ARBs: Candesartan 4 mg PO daily (usual 8–32 mg); Losartan 25 mg PO daily (25–100 mg)
- DHP-CCB: Amlodipine 2.5 mg PO daily (titrate to 5–10 mg)
- Avoid alpha-blockers and centrally acting agents for routine therapy (orthostasis, CNS effects)

Complications / Prognosis

- Poor control: stroke, MI, HF, CKD progression
- Over-treatment: falls, syncope, AKI
- With individualized control: reduced cardiovascular events and improved safety

Red Flags (When to Escalate/Transfer)

- Hypertensive emergency (BP $\geq$180/120 with acute end-organ damage)
- Refractory orthostatic hypotension with syncope/falls
- Rapid creatinine rise or hyperkalemia after RAAS initiation

Prevention / Health Promotion

- Regular seated/standing BP checks; medication reviews
- Vaccination (influenza, pneumococcal) to reduce CV complications
- Encourage activity and low-sodium diets in LTC menus

References (Open-Access)

- NICE Guideline – Hypertension in adults (NG136): https://www.nice.org.uk/guidance/ng136
- NHS – High blood pressure (hypertension): https://www.nhs.uk/conditions/high-blood-pressure-hypertension/
- Public Health Agency of Canada – Heart health: https://www.canada.ca/en/public-health

CHAPTER 14
Heart Failure in LTC

Overview

Heart failure (HF) is common in LTC and presents with dyspnea, edema, and fatigue. Management focuses on symptom relief, preventing hospitalizations, and evidence-based therapy adapted for frailty and renal function. Differentiate HFrEF (reduced EF) and HFpEF (preserved EF).

Risk Factors / Epidemiology

- Ischemic heart disease, long-standing hypertension
- Valvular disease, atrial fibrillation
- Diabetes, CKD, obesity, COPD
- Advanced age with multimorbidity

Clinical Presentation

- Dyspnea on exertion or at rest, orthopnea, PND
- Peripheral edema, weight gain, fatigue
- Crackles, elevated JVP, S3 (HFrEF) or hypertension/LAE (HFpEF)

Assessment / Investigations

- Vitals, weight, volume status (daily weights when decompensated)
- Labs: BMP (Na/K/Cr), eGFR, BNP/NT-proBNP if available; LFTs
- ECG (AF, ischemia), CXR (pulmonary edema), echocardiogram to classify EF if feasible
- Review precipitating factors (infection, anemia, arrhythmia, high salt intake, NSAIDs)

Management

Non-pharmacological:

- Sodium restriction (e.g., 2 g/day) and fluid restriction if hyponatremic
- Daily weights; educate to report >1–2 kg gain in 2–3 days
- Moderate activity as tolerated; elevate legs for edema
- Vaccinations; avoid NSAIDs; review medications for negative inotropes

Pharmacological (start low, go slow; monitor BP, K+, Cr):

- **Loop diuretics:** Furosemide 20–40 mg PO daily (titrate to symptoms); Torsemide 5–10 mg PO daily
- ACEi/ARB: Lisinopril 2.5–5 mg PO daily (goal 20–40 mg); Valsartan 40 mg PO BID (up to 160 mg BID)
- **ARNI:** Sacubitril/Valsartan 24/26 mg PO BID (titrate to 49/51 mg BID then 97/103 mg BID if tolerated; washout 36h after ACEi)
- **Beta-blockers (HFrEF):** Bisoprolol 1.25 mg PO daily; Metoprolol succinate 12.5–25 mg PO daily; Carvedilol 3.125 mg PO BID
- **MRA:** Spironolactone 12.5–25 mg PO daily (monitor K+, Cr; avoid if K+>5.0 or eGFR <30)
- **SGLT2 inhibitors:** Dapagliflozin 10 mg PO daily or Empagliflozin 10 mg PO daily (benefit in HFrEF/HFpEF; check renal function)
- **HFpEF focus:** Control BP, diuretics for congestion, SGLT2 inhibitor; manage AF and ischemia

Complications / Prognosis

- Recurrent decompensation, renal dysfunction, hyperkalemia
- Arrhythmias, thromboembolism, frequent hospitalizations
- Prognosis varies; careful titration improves quality of life and reduces admissions

Red Flags (When to Escalate/Transfer)

- Severe dyspnea at rest, hypoxia, pulmonary edema
- Rapid weight gain with refractory edema despite diuretics
- Hyperkalemia, acute kidney injury, symptomatic hypotension
- Suspected ACS or rapid AF with hemodynamic compromise

Prevention / Health Promotion

- Vaccinations (influenza, pneumococcal), sodium-aware menus
- Medication reconciliation and avoidance of NSAIDs
- Early recognition protocols for fluid overload in LTC

References (Open-Access)

- NICE Guideline – Chronic heart failure in adults (NG106): https://www.nice.org.uk/guidance/ng106
- NHS – Heart failure overview: https://www.nhs.uk/conditions/heart-failure/
- Public Health Agency of Canada – Heart disease: https://www.canada.ca/en/public-health

CHAPTER 15
Atrial Fibrillation & Anticoagulation

Overview

Atrial fibrillation (AF) is common in LTC and increases the risk of stroke and heart failure. Management includes stroke prevention with anticoagulation, rate control, and symptom management.

Risk Factors / Epidemiology

- Age, hypertension, heart failure, valvular disease
- Diabetes, obesity, sleep apnea, hyperthyroidism
- Prior stroke/TIA, CKD
- Polypharmacy and frailty influence bleeding risk

Clinical Presentation

- Palpitations, dyspnea, fatigue; may be asymptomatic
- Irregularly irregular pulse; tachycardia
- Dizziness, syncope in rapid ventricular response

Assessment / Investigations

- ECG to confirm AF; rate/rhythm; consider echocardiogram if feasible
- CHA_2DS_2-VASc for stroke risk; HAS-BLED for bleeding risk (guide but do not deny anticoagulation solely on score)
- Labs: CBC, renal/hepatic function, TSH; review drugs (NSAIDs, antiplatelets)

Management

Non-pharmacological:

- Discuss goals of care and fall risk mitigation
- Manage triggers (thyrotoxicosis, infection, alcohol), treat sleep apnea
- Rate control preferred in LTC; rhythm control rarely indicated unless highly symptomatic

Pharmacological:

- -Anticoagulation (typical doses; adjust for renal function/age/weight):
- Apixaban 5 mg PO BID (reduce to 2.5 mg BID if ≥2 of: age ≥80, weight ≤60 kg, serum creatinine ≥133 μmol/L/1.5 mg/dL)
- Rivaroxaban 20 mg PO daily with food (15 mg daily if CrCl 15–50 mL/min)
- Dabigatran 150 mg PO BID (110 mg BID if age ≥80 or high bleed risk; avoid if CrCl <30)
- Edoxaban 60 mg PO daily (30 mg daily if CrCl 15–50 mL/min or weight ≤60 kg)
- Warfarin: start 2–5 mg PO daily; target INR 2–3; frequent monitoring; fewer interactions preferred in LTC when stable
- Rate control: Metoprolol succinate 12.5–25 mg PO daily (titrate); Bisoprolol 1.25 mg PO daily; Diltiazem CD 120 mg PO daily (avoid in HFrEF); Digoxin 0.0625–0.125 mg PO daily (monitor levels/renal function)
- Avoid routine dual therapy (anticoagulant + antiplatelet) unless recent ACS/stent per cardiology

Complications / Prognosis

- Ischemic stroke, systemic embolism
- Bleeding (GI, intracranial) – risk mitigated by correct dosing and PPI if needed
- Tachycardia-induced cardiomyopathy if uncontrolled rate

Red Flags (When to Escalate/Transfer)

- Hemodynamic instability, chest pain, syncope
- New neurologic deficits (suspected stroke/TIA)
- GI bleed, melena, or major bleeding on anticoagulant

Prevention / Health Promotion

- Blood pressure control, weight management, sleep apnea treatment
- Avoid excess alcohol; smoking cessation
- Adherence support and regular renal function checks for DOAC dosing

References (Open-Access)

- NICE Guideline – Atrial fibrillation (NG196): https://www.nice.org.uk/guidance/ng196
- Thrombosis Canada – Atrial Fibrillation & Anticoagulation Guides: https://thrombosiscanada.ca
- NHS – Atrial fibrillation overview: https://www.nhs.uk/conditions/atrial-fibrillation/

CHAPTER 16
Peripheral Vascular Disease (Peripheral Arterial Disease – PAD)

Overview

Peripheral arterial disease (PAD) is a manifestation of systemic atherosclerosis causing reduced blood flow to the limbs. In LTC it presents with claudication, rest pain, non-healing ulcers, and is a marker of high CV risk.

Risk Factors / Epidemiology

- Age, smoking, diabetes, hypertension, dyslipidemia
- CKD, obesity, sedentary lifestyle
- Coexistent CAD and cerebrovascular disease common

Clinical Presentation

- Intermittent claudication (calf pain with walking, relieved by rest)
- Rest pain, cool/pale extremities, hair loss, thickened nails
- Diminished/absent pulses; non-healing ulcers or gangrene in severe disease

Assessment / Investigations

- Vascular exam (pulses, bruits, skin integrity); foot inspection each visit
- Ankle–brachial index (ABI) if available (PAD likely if ≤0.90)
- Labs: lipids, A1c/glucose, renal function

- Consider duplex ultrasound if critical limb-threatening ischemia suspected

Management

Non-pharmacological:

- Supervised or structured walking programs (walk to moderate pain, rest, repeat)
- Smoking cessation support; foot care education and protective footwear
- Optimize diabetes, BP, and lipid control

Pharmacological:

- **Antiplatelet:** Clopidogrel 75 mg PO daily preferred; or Aspirin 75–81 mg PO daily if clopidogrel not tolerated
- **Lipid-lowering:** Atorvastatin 20–40 mg PO daily (consider 80 mg if tolerated); or Rosuvastatin 10–20 mg PO daily
- **ACE inhibitor/ARB:** Perindopril 2–4 mg PO daily (CV risk reduction)
- **Cilostazol:** 100 mg PO BID for claudication (avoid in heart failure)
- **Dual pathway in select high-risk:** Rivaroxaban 2.5 mg PO BID + Aspirin 81 mg PO daily (consider bleeding risk; specialist input)

Complications / Prognosis

- Critical limb-threatening ischemia, infection, amputation
- High risk of MI and stroke
- Exercise therapy and risk-factor control improve walking distance and outcomes

Red Flags (When to Escalate/Transfer)

- Acute limb ischemia (sudden pain, pallor, pulselessness, paralysis, paresthesia, poikilothermia)
- Spreading infection, wet gangrene, or deep ulcers
- Severe rest pain unresponsive to initial measures

Prevention / Health Promotion

- Smoking cessation; daily foot checks; appropriate footwear
- BP, lipid, and glucose targets individualized for frailty
- Vaccinations and exercise programs in LTC

References (Open-Access)

- NICE Guideline – Peripheral arterial disease (CG147): https://www.nice.org.uk/guidance/cg147
- NHS – Peripheral arterial disease: https://www.nhs.uk/conditions/peripheral-arterial-disease-pad/
- Public Health Agency of Canada – Atherosclerosis: https://www.canada.ca/en/public-health

C.) MEDICAL CONDITIONS COMMON IN LTC – RESPIRATORY

CHAPTER 17
Chronic Obstructive Pulmonary Disease (COPD) Management

Overview

COPD is a progressive lung disease characterized by airflow limitation that is not fully reversible. In LTC, many residents present with advanced disease, frequent exacerbations, and functional impairment. Management focuses on symptom control, preventing exacerbations, optimizing quality of life, and advance care planning.

Risk Factors / Epidemiology

- Smoking history (primary risk factor)
- Occupational exposures (dust, chemicals)
- Age >65 years
- Recurrent respiratory infections
- Low socioeconomic status and limited access to healthcare

Clinical Presentation

- Chronic cough, sputum production, exertional dyspnea
- Wheeze, prolonged expiratory phase
- Exacerbations: increased cough, sputum purulence/volume, dyspnea
- Advanced disease: hypoxemia, hypercapnia, cachexia, cor pulmonale

Assessment / Investigations

- Diagnosis: spirometry (FEV1/FVC <0.7 post-bronchodilator) – often unavailable in LTC; rely on clinical history
- Pulse oximetry (target SpO2 88–92% in severe COPD)
- CXR to exclude pneumonia or other pathology
- Labs: CBC (polycythemia), ABG if severe
- Review triggers: infection, CHF, medication non-adherence

Management

Non-pharmacological:

- Smoking cessation support
- Vaccinations: influenza, pneumococcal, COVID-19
- Pulmonary rehabilitation or physiotherapy (if feasible)
- Nutritional support for cachexia; palliative approach in end-stage disease

Pharmacological:

1. **Bronchodilators:**
   - **Short-acting:** Salbutamol 100 mcg (1–2 puffs q4–6h PRN); Ipratropium 20 mcg (2 puffs QID)
   - **Long-acting:** Tiotropium 18 mcg inhaled once daily; Formoterol 12 mcg BID; Salmeterol 50 mcg BID
2. **Combination inhalers:** LAMA/LABA or LABA/ICS for frequent exacerbations
3. **Oral corticosteroids for exacerbations:** Prednisone 40 mg PO daily × 5 days
4. **Antibiotics if infectious exacerbation with increased sputum purulence:**

- Amoxicillin-clavulanate 875/125 mg PO BID × 5–7 days
- Doxycycline 100 mg PO BID × 5–7 days (if penicillin allergy)
5 **Oxygen therapy:** indicated if chronic hypoxemia (PaO2 ≤55 mmHg or SpO2 ≤88%)
6 **Avoid routine use:** Theophylline, chronic oral steroids

Complications / Prognosis

- Exacerbations → hospitalizations, functional decline
- Cor pulmonale, respiratory failure, cachexia
- Prognosis varies with GOLD stage and comorbidities

Red Flags (When to Escalate/Transfer)

- Severe dyspnea unresponsive to initial therapy
- Hypoxemia (SpO2 <85%) or hypercapnic encephalopathy
- Suspected pneumonia, PE, or pneumothorax
- Need for non-invasive ventilation or ICU

Prevention / Health Promotion

- Smoking cessation programs
- Regular vaccinations
- Avoid exposure to indoor/outdoor pollutants
- Pulmonary rehab and physical activity encouragement

References (Open-Access)

- NHS – COPD overview: https://www.nhs.uk/conditions/chronic-obstructive-pulmonary-disease-copd/
- Public Health Agency of Canada – COPD: https://www.canada.ca/en/public-health/services/chronic-diseases/chronic-obstructive-pulmonary-disease.html
- Global Initiative for Chronic Obstructive Lung Disease (GOLD) – Strategy Report (free PDF): https://goldcopd.org

CHAPTER 18
Aspiration Pneumonia & Dysphagia

Overview

Aspiration pneumonia occurs when oropharyngeal or gastric contents are inhaled into the lungs, leading to infection. It is common in frail LTC residents with dysphagia, neurologic disease, or poor oral hygiene. Prevention and early management are critical to reduce morbidity and mortality.

Risk Factors / Epidemiology

- Dementia, Parkinson's disease, stroke
- Dysphagia from neuromuscular disease or frailty
- Poor dentition and oral hygiene
- Sedatives, opioids, antipsychotics (reduce protective reflexes)
- Tube feeding (risk of aspiration of gastric contents)

Clinical Presentation

- Cough, fever, dyspnea, purulent sputum
- Tachypnea, hypoxemia, crackles
- Delirium or functional decline may be first sign in elderly
- Often right lower lobe infiltrates on CXR

Assessment / Investigations

- Clinical history (choking, witnessed aspiration)
- Physical exam: fever, hypoxemia, lung findings
- CXR (infiltrates, aspiration pattern)
- CBC, CRP; cultures if severe

- Swallowing assessment by SLP if recurrent

Management

Non-pharmacological:

- Elevate head of bed 30–45° during and after meals
- Swallowing therapy and texture-modified diets
- Oral hygiene protocols in LTC
- Minimize sedative/anticholinergic use
- Advance care planning in recurrent aspiration cases

Pharmacological:

1. **Empiric antibiotics (consider local resistance):**
   - Amoxicillin-clavulanate 875/125 mg PO BID × 5–7 days
   - Ceftriaxone 1 g IV daily × 5–7 days (if more severe)
   - Alternatives: Doxycycline 100 mg PO BID × 5–7 days; Levofloxacin 500 mg PO daily × 5 days
2. Avoid clindamycin unless anaerobic infection strongly suspected (↑ C. difficile risk)
3. Supplemental oxygen if hypoxemic; bronchodilators if COPD/asthma overlap

Complications / Prognosis

- Respiratory failure, sepsis
- Recurrent aspiration → chronic lung disease
- High mortality in frail elderly
- Prevention strategies essential to reduce recurrence

Red Flags (When to Escalate/Transfer)

- Severe hypoxemia or respiratory distress
- Sepsis or hemodynamic instability

- Failure to improve with initial oral therapy
- Consider hospitalization if unable to maintain oral intake or high aspiration risk

Prevention / Health Promotion

- Routine swallowing assessments in high-risk residents
- Oral hygiene protocols (brushing teeth twice daily)
- Positioning strategies and supervised feeding
- ACP discussions for residents with recurrent aspiration

References (Open-Access)

- NHS – Aspiration pneumonia: https://www.nhs.uk/conditions/aspiration-pneumonia/
- Public Health Agency of Canada – Pneumonia: https://www.canada.ca/en/public-health/services/diseases/pneumonia.html
- Infection Prevention and Control Canada: https://ipac-canada.org

CHAPTER 19
Oxygen Therapy in Long-Term Care

Overview

Oxygen therapy in LTC is used for residents with chronic hypoxemia, usually from COPD, heart failure, or interstitial lung disease. It improves survival in chronic hypoxemia, relieves dyspnea, and enhances quality of life. Indications, monitoring, and safety are critical.

Risk Factors / Epidemiology

- Chronic lung disease (COPD, interstitial lung disease)
- Heart failure with hypoxemia
- Recurrent pneumonia or pulmonary fibrosis
- Older age and frailty increase risk of oxygen dependence

Clinical Presentation

- Dyspnea on exertion or at rest
- Fatigue, confusion, cyanosis
- Clubbing in chronic hypoxemia
- Documented low SpO2 or PaO2

Assessment / Investigations

- Pulse oximetry (room air, at rest and exertion)
- ABG if severe COPD or suspected CO2 retention
- CXR, ECG, echo if differential includes CHF
- Functional assessment (6-min walk, if feasible)

Management

Non-pharmacological:

- Smoking cessation and pulmonary rehab when possible
- Positioning for dyspnea (tripod, forward leaning)
- Breathing exercises (pursed lip, diaphragmatic)
- Ensure equipment safety (no smoking near oxygen)
- ACP for residents requiring continuous oxygen

Pharmacological:

1. **Indications for LTOT:**
   - PaO_2 ≤55 mmHg or SpO_2 ≤88% at rest on room air
   - PaO_2 56–59 mmHg with cor pulmonale, right heart failure, or hematocrit >55%
2. **Dosing:** Titrate to SpO_2 88–92% in COPD; 90–94% in other chronic hypoxemia
3. **Devices:** Nasal cannula preferred; 1–6 L/min (FiO_2 approx. 24–44%)
4. **Monitoring:** Check SpO_2 regularly, reassess need every 6–12 months; monitor for CO_2 retention in COPD
5. **Avoid over-oxygenation:** In severe COPD, high O_2 can worsen hypercapnia

Complications / Prognosis

- Nasal dryness, epistaxis, skin breakdown
- Fire hazard with smoking
- CO_2 retention in COPD if excessive O_2 given
- LTOT improves survival in severe chronic hypoxemia; improves exercise tolerance and sleep quality

Red Flags (When to Escalate/Transfer)

- Severe respiratory distress unresponsive to oxygen
- Hypercapnic encephalopathy (confusion, somnolence)
- Refractory hypoxemia despite high-flow O2
- Sudden desaturation suggesting PE, pneumothorax, pneumonia

Prevention / Health Promotion

- Regular reassessment of oxygen requirement
- Vaccinations (influenza, pneumococcal, COVID-19)
- Smoking cessation programs in LTC
- Education of staff and families on oxygen safety

References (Open-Access)

- NHS – Oxygen therapy: https://www.nhs.uk/conditions/oxygen-therapy/
- British Thoracic Society – Home oxygen guideline (open access): https://www.brit-thoracic.org.uk
- Public Health Agency of Canada – COPD and lung disease: https://www.canada.ca/en/public-health

D.) MEDICAL CONDITIONS COMMON IN LTC – ENDOCRINE / METABOLIC

CHAPTER 20
Diabetes Management in Elderly

Overview

Diabetes mellitus is common in LTC and associated with complications such as hypoglycemia, infections, cardiovascular disease, and functional decline. In frail elderly, management emphasizes symptom control, avoidance of hypoglycemia, and individualized targets rather than strict glycemic control.

Risk Factors / Epidemiology

- Prevalence increases with age; common in LTC populations
- Obesity, physical inactivity, family history
- Ethnic predisposition (Indigenous, South Asian, African descent)
- Polypharmacy, multimorbidity, limited life expectancy

Clinical Presentation

- May be asymptomatic; often diagnosed via routine labs
- Polyuria, polydipsia, nocturia
- Fatigue, weight loss, recurrent infections (UTI, skin)
- Hypoglycemia may present as confusion, falls, or delirium

Assessment / Investigations

- Fasting glucose, HbA1c (interpret cautiously in frailty/anemia)
- Urinalysis for proteinuria; eGFR for renal dosing
- Lipid panel, BP, weight

- Screen for complications: foot exams, neuropathy, retinopathy (as feasible in LTC)

Management

Non-pharmacological:

- **Individualize glycemic targets:** HbA1c 7.5–8.5% in frail elderly; focus on avoiding hypoglycemia
- Balanced diet, consistent meal timing, avoid restrictive diets in underweight residents
- Encourage gentle physical activity if safe
- Foot care and regular skin inspections

Pharmacological:

- **Metformin:** 500 mg PO daily, titrate to 1000 mg BID; avoid if eGFR <30 mL/min; reduce dose if eGFR 30–45
- **DPP-4 inhibitors (e.g., Sitagliptin):** 100 mg PO daily; reduce to 25–50 mg daily if eGFR <50
- **SGLT2 inhibitors (e.g., Empagliflozin 10 mg PO daily):** benefits in CV and renal outcomes; avoid if eGFR <30
- **Sulfonylureas:** Avoid glyburide; if needed, use gliclazide MR 30 mg PO daily; monitor hypoglycemia risk
- **Insulin:** If required, use basal insulin (glargine or detemir 5–10 units HS); titrate cautiously; avoid complex regimens in frail elderly
- Avoid TZDs (fluid retention, fractures) and aggressive insulin regimens in LTC

Complications / Prognosis

- Hypoglycemia, falls, delirium
- Infections, poor wound healing
- Macrovascular disease (MI, stroke)
- With appropriate targets: improved comfort, reduced hospitalizations

Red Flags (When to Escalate/Transfer)

- Severe hypoglycemia (unconsciousness, seizures)
- Hyperglycemic crisis (DKA, HHS)
- Rapid decline in renal function or new foot ulcer/infection

Prevention / Health Promotion

- Regular foot care and skin checks
- Vaccinations (influenza, pneumococcal)
- Staff education on recognizing hypoglycemia
- Simplified medication regimens and deprescribing where possible

References (Open-Access)

- Diabetes Canada – Clinical Practice Guidelines (open access summaries): https://guidelines.diabetes.ca
- Public Health Agency of Canada – Diabetes: https://www.canada.ca/en/public-health/services/chronic-diseases/diabetes.html
- World Health Organization – Diabetes Fact Sheet: https://www.who.int/news-room/fact-sheets/detail/diabetes

CHAPTER 21
Thyroid Disorders in Elderly

Overview

Thyroid disorders are common in LTC residents, especially hypothyroidism and less commonly hyperthyroidism. Symptoms may be subtle and mimic aging or dementia. Care must be taken to avoid overtreatment due to cardiac and bone risks.

Risk Factors / Epidemiology

- Advanced age, female sex
- Autoimmune thyroid disease (Hashimoto's, Graves')
- Prior neck irradiation or surgery
- Amiodarone or lithium therapy
- Iodine deficiency/excess

Clinical Presentation

- Hypothyroidism: fatigue, weight gain, constipation, dry skin, cold intolerance, cognitive decline
- Hyperthyroidism: weight loss, heat intolerance, tremor, palpitations, atrial fibrillation
- Subclinical disease common in elderly; may present as apathy, depression, or functional decline

Assessment / Investigations

- TSH, free T4
- Lipids, CBC (macrocytosis in hypothyroidism)
- ECG for AF in hyperthyroidism
- Thyroid antibodies if autoimmune suspected

Management

Hypothyroidism:

- Levothyroxine: start low (12.5–25 mcg PO daily) in frail elderly; titrate q6–8 weeks to target TSH 4–6 (slightly higher than younger adults)
- Monitor for angina, arrhythmia, osteoporosis
- Avoid overtreatment (TSH <0.5)

Hyperthyroidism:

- If Graves' disease/toxic nodules: Endocrinology referral if possible
- Beta-blocker for symptoms: Propranolol 10–20 mg PO TID or Metoprolol 12.5–25 mg PO BID
- Antithyroid drugs: Methimazole 2.5–5 mg PO daily in elderly (use lowest dose to normalize TSH; monitor CBC/LFTs)
- Avoid overtreatment; target euthyroid state

Complications / Prognosis

- Hypothyroidism: cognitive impairment, depression, bradycardia, constipation, falls
- Hyperthyroidism: AF, osteoporosis, heart failure, delirium
- Good prognosis with cautious treatment and monitoring

Red Flags (When to Escalate/Transfer)

- Severe hypothyroidism (myxedema coma)
- Thyrotoxic crisis (thyroid storm): fever, tachyarrhythmia, delirium

- Chest pain, new AF, or acute heart failure during therapy adjustment

Prevention / Health Promotion

- Regular TSH monitoring in elderly with non-specific symptoms
- Avoid excess iodine or unnecessary thyroid supplements
- Monitor carefully when adjusting levothyroxine in elderly

References (Open-Access)

- NHS – Underactive thyroid: https://www.nhs.uk/conditions/underactive-thyroid-hypothyroidism/
- NHS – Overactive thyroid: https://www.nhs.uk/conditions/overactive-thyroid-hyperthyroidism/
- Public Health Agency of Canada – Thyroid disease overview: https://www.canada.ca/en/public-health

CHAPTER 22
Osteoporosis & Fracture Prevention

Overview

Osteoporosis is common in LTC and leads to fragility fractures, particularly hip fractures, which are associated with high morbidity and mortality. Prevention and treatment strategies reduce fracture risk and preserve mobility.

Risk Factors / Epidemiology

- Advanced age, female sex
- Low BMI, poor nutrition, vitamin D deficiency
- Sedentary lifestyle, smoking, alcohol use
- Medications: glucocorticoids, PPIs, anticonvulsants
- Dementia, falls, prior fractures

Clinical Presentation

- Often silent until fracture occurs
- Vertebral compression fractures: back pain, kyphosis, height loss
- Hip fracture: acute pain, inability to bear weight
- Functional decline and immobility

Assessment / Investigations

- Clinical diagnosis often in LTC after fragility fracture
- Bone mineral density (DEXA) if available, though often impractical in LTC
- Labs: calcium, phosphate, vitamin D, renal and liver function, TSH if secondary causes suspected

Management

Non-pharmacological:

- Fall prevention: strength/balance training, mobility aids, safe environment
- Adequate calcium intake: 1000–1200 mg/day (diet + supplements)
- Vitamin D supplementation: 800–1000 IU daily (higher if deficiency)
- Hip protectors in LTC; encourage weight-bearing activity

Pharmacological:

- **Bisphosphonates:** Alendronate 70 mg PO weekly or Risedronate 35 mg PO weekly; avoid if eGFR <30
- **IV bisphosphonate:** Zoledronic acid 5 mg IV yearly (if eGFR >35)
- **Denosumab:** 60 mg SC q6 months; safe in renal impairment but requires calcium/vitamin D supplementation
- **Raloxifene:** 60 mg PO daily (selective use in women; avoid with VTE risk)
- **Hormone therapy:** generally avoided in elderly due to risks

Complications / Prognosis

- Fragility fractures (hip, vertebral, wrist)
- Functional decline, loss of independence, chronic pain
- Mortality risk high after hip fracture
- Prevention and treatment significantly reduce fracture risk

Red Flags (When to Escalate/Transfer)

- New hip or vertebral fracture
- Severe or refractory back pain
- Hypocalcemia with bisphosphonate or denosumab therapy
- Suspected osteonecrosis of the jaw (rare)

Prevention / Health Promotion

- Universal vitamin D and calcium supplementation in LTC
- Regular exercise and fall prevention programs
- Medication review to minimize fall risk
- Early mobilization post-fracture to preserve function

References (Open-Access)

- Osteoporosis Canada – Guidelines and resources: https://osteoporosis.ca
- Public Health Agency of Canada – Osteoporosis: https://www.canada.ca/en/public-health/services/chronic-diseases/osteoporosis.html
- NHS – Osteoporosis overview: https://www.nhs.uk/conditions/osteoporosis/

E.) MEDICAL CONDITIONS COMMON IN LTC – RENAL / GENITOURINARY (GU)

CHAPTER 23
Chronic Kidney Disease (CKD) in Elderly

Overview

CKD is common in older adults due to hypertension, diabetes, and vascular disease. In LTC, management emphasizes slowing progression, preventing complications, and avoiding nephrotoxic drugs. Dialysis is rarely initiated in frail elderly; conservative management is often more appropriate.

Risk Factors / Epidemiology

- Hypertension, diabetes, cardiovascular disease
- Advanced age, frailty, polypharmacy
- Recurrent UTIs, nephrotoxic drugs (NSAIDs, contrast agents)
- Proteinuria and family history of CKD

Clinical Presentation

- Often asymptomatic until advanced stage
- Fatigue, anorexia, pruritus, nocturia
- Volume overload (edema, hypertension)
- Cognitive changes in advanced disease

Assessment / Investigations

- Labs: serum creatinine, eGFR, electrolytes, calcium, phosphate, hemoglobin, albumin
- Urinalysis and albumin-creatinine ratio (ACR)
- BP monitoring; review meds for nephrotoxins
- Renal ultrasound if obstruction suspected

Management

Non-pharmacological:

- Optimize BP and diabetes control
- Avoid dehydration and nephrotoxic drugs (NSAIDs, contrast)
- Dietary advice: moderate protein and salt restriction
- ACP discussions in advanced CKD

Pharmacological:

- ACE inhibitors/ARBs (e.g., Perindopril 2–4 mg PO daily; Losartan 25 mg PO daily) for proteinuric CKD
- Diuretics for volume overload (e.g., Furosemide 20–40 mg PO daily; titrate as needed)
- Erythropoiesis-stimulating agents rarely used in LTC; consider only if symptomatic anemia and specialist input
- Adjust drug doses to renal function (e.g., antibiotics, hypoglycemics)
- Avoid routine phosphate binders unless specialist advised

Complications / Prognosis

- Anemia, electrolyte disorders (hyperkalemia, acidosis)
- Fluid overload, heart failure
- Increased infection risk
- Poor prognosis with advanced CKD in frail elderly; conservative care often appropriate

Red Flags (When to Escalate/Transfer)

- Rapid decline in eGFR or acute kidney injury
- Hyperkalemia >6.0 mmol/L
- Severe volume overload unresponsive to diuretics
- Symptomatic uremia (confusion, pericarditis, seizures)

References (Open-Access)

- NHS – Chronic kidney disease:
  https://www.nhs.uk/conditions/kidney-disease/
- Public Health Agency of Canada – Kidney health:
  https://www.canada.ca/en/public-health
- National Kidney Foundation (patient resources):
  https://www.kidney.org

CHAPTER 24
Urinary Incontinence

Overview

Urinary incontinence is highly prevalent in LTC residents and contributes to falls, skin breakdown, infections, and reduced quality of life. It is often multifactorial and requires a comprehensive assessment before treatment.

Risk Factors / Epidemiology

- Advanced age, female sex
- Dementia, Parkinson's, stroke, mobility limitations
- Diabetes, chronic cough, constipation
- Medications: diuretics, sedatives, anticholinergics

Clinical Presentation

- Stress incontinence: leakage with cough, laugh, exertion
- Urge incontinence: sudden urge with leakage
- Overflow: dribbling, incomplete emptying (often BPH in men)
- Functional: inability to reach toilet due to mobility/cognitive issues

Assessment / Investigations

- History, bladder diary, review medications
- Physical exam: abdomen, pelvic/prostate exam if feasible
- Urinalysis to exclude UTI
- Post-void residual (ultrasound or bladder scan)

Management

Non-pharmacological:

- Toileting schedules, prompted voiding
- Pelvic floor exercises (if able)
- Reduce caffeine/alcohol; manage constipation
- Absorbent products as supportive measure

Pharmacological:

- Urge incontinence: Oxybutynin 2.5 mg PO BID (use lowest dose; avoid in frail elderly due to anticholinergic effects)
- Alternatives: Mirabegron 25 mg PO daily (monitor BP; avoid if uncontrolled hypertension)
- Stress incontinence: limited pharmacological options; duloxetine rarely used in elderly
- Overflow incontinence: address obstruction (see BPH)

References (Open-Access)

- NHS – Urinary incontinence: https://www.nhs.uk/conditions/urinary-incontinence/
- Public Health Agency of Canada – Bladder health: https://www.canada.ca/en/public-health
- Canadian Continence Foundation: https://www.canadiancontinence.ca

CHAPTER 25
Benign Prostatic Hyperplasia (BPH)

Overview

BPH is a common cause of lower urinary tract symptoms in elderly men. In LTC, treatment focuses on symptom relief, preventing retention, and avoiding polypharmacy complications.

Risk Factors / Epidemiology

- Age >60 years
- Family history, obesity, metabolic syndrome
- Medications: anticholinergics, opioids, antihistamines may worsen symptoms

Clinical Presentation

- Lower urinary tract symptoms (LUTS): hesitancy, weak stream, nocturia, incomplete emptying
- Acute urinary retention
- Recurrent UTIs or bladder stones in severe obstruction

Assessment / Investigations

- History and International Prostate Symptom Score (IPSS) if feasible
- DRE if appropriate
- Urinalysis, creatinine (if chronic obstruction suspected)
- Post-void residual with bladder scan

Management

Non-pharmacological:

- Avoid evening fluids, caffeine, alcohol
- Scheduled toileting, double voiding
- Review medications that worsen LUTS

Pharmacological:

- Alpha-blockers: Tamsulosin 0.4 mg PO daily (monitor orthostasis, falls)
- 5-alpha-reductase inhibitors: Finasteride 5 mg PO daily (takes 6–12 months for effect)
- Combination therapy if severe symptoms and prostate enlarged
- Avoid anticholinergics in frail elderly due to delirium risk

References (Open-Access)

- NHS – Enlarged prostate (BPH): https://www.nhs.uk/conditions/prostate-enlargement/
- Public Health Agency of Canada – Prostate health: https://www.canada.ca/en/public-health
- Canadian Urological Association – Patient resources: https://www.cua.org

CHAPTER 26
Recurrent Urinary Tract Infections (UTIs)

Overview

Recurrent UTIs are common in LTC residents, particularly women, those with catheters, and individuals with incontinence or poor hygiene. Prevention strategies are central; indiscriminate antibiotic use should be avoided to reduce resistance and C. difficile risk.

Risk Factors / Epidemiology

- Female sex, postmenopausal estrogen deficiency
- Dementia, incontinence, immobility
- Catheter use, incomplete emptying (e.g., BPH)
- Diabetes, poor perineal hygiene

Clinical Presentation

- Dysuria, frequency, urgency, suprapubic pain
- In elderly, may present with delirium, falls, or functional decline
- Fever, flank pain if upper tract involvement
- Must distinguish asymptomatic bacteriuria (do not treat)

Assessment / Investigations

Urinalysis and urine culture if symptomatic

- Avoid routine screening/treatment of asymptomatic bacteriuria except in pregnancy or prior to urologic procedures
- Assess for post-void residual and contributing factors

Management

Non-pharmacological:

- Hydration and toileting programs
- Perineal hygiene; avoid unnecessary catheters
- Topical vaginal estrogen for postmenopausal women (e.g., estradiol 10 mcg PV 2–3x/week)
- Cranberry extract (limited evidence)
- Probiotics under study; evidence limited

Pharmacological:

- Acute UTI: Nitrofurantoin 100 mg PO BID × 5 days (avoid if eGFR <30)
- TMP-SMX 1 DS PO BID × 3 days (avoid if resistance >20% locally)
- Fosfomycin 3 g PO single dose
- Prophylaxis (selected residents with ≥3 UTIs/year): Nitrofurantoin 50–100 mg PO HS; or TMP-SMX SS PO HS
- Rotate or reassess prophylaxis q6–12 months to limit resistance

References (Open-Access)

- NHS – Urinary tract infections (UTIs): https://www.nhs.uk/conditions/urinary-tract-infections-utis/
- Public Health Agency of Canada – UTIs: https://www.canada.ca/en/public-health
- Infection Prevention and Control Canada: https://ipac-canada.org

F.) MEDICAL CONDITIONS COMMON IN LTC – GASTROINTESTINAL / NUTRITION

CHAPTER 26
Dysphagia & Aspiration Risk

Overview

Dysphagia is difficulty swallowing, common in LTC residents due to stroke, Parkinson's disease, dementia, or frailty. It increases the risk of aspiration pneumonia, malnutrition, and dehydration. Management emphasizes safe swallowing strategies and individualized nutrition support.

Risk Factors / Epidemiology

- Neurologic disease (stroke, dementia, Parkinson's, ALS)
- Frailty, poor dentition, decreased consciousness
- Sedatives, antipsychotics, or opioids
- Advanced age and multimorbidity

Clinical Presentation

- Coughing or choking with meals
- Wet or gurgly voice
- Recurrent pneumonia, unexplained weight loss
- Pocketing food, prolonged mealtime
- Dehydration, malnutrition

Assessment / Investigations

- Bedside swallowing assessment by nursing/SLP
- Videofluoroscopic swallow study (VFSS) if available
- Nutritional assessment (weight, BMI, labs)
- Oral exam for dentition and hygiene

Management

Non-pharmacological:

- Texture-modified diets (pureed, minced, thickened liquids)
- Upright posture during and after meals (30–45 min)
- Small bites, slow pace, supervised feeding
- Oral hygiene after meals
- Feeding tubes: consider goals of care; not always beneficial in advanced dementia

Pharmacological:

- No direct medications for dysphagia; avoid sedatives/anticholinergics that worsen swallowing
- Treat underlying conditions (e.g., optimize Parkinson's therapy)

References (Open-Access)

- NHS – Swallowing difficulties (dysphagia): https://www.nhs.uk/conditions/swallowing-problems-dysphagia/
- Public Health Agency of Canada – Seniors and Nutrition: https://www.canada.ca/en/public-health
- Canadian Society of Nutrition Management: https://csnm.in1touch.org

CHAPTER 27
Malnutrition & Weight Loss

Overview

Malnutrition is common in LTC and associated with frailty, infections, pressure ulcers, and mortality. Causes include poor intake, swallowing difficulty, chronic illness, and depression. Prevention and management focus on screening, nutrition support, and addressing reversible factors.

Risk Factors / Epidemiology

- Dementia, depression, swallowing disorders
- Poor dentition, ill-fitting dentures
- Chronic diseases (CKD, COPD, cancer)
- Polypharmacy, anorexia-inducing drugs
- Social isolation, limited assistance with feeding

Clinical Presentation

- Unintentional weight loss (>5% in 6 months)
- Low BMI (<18.5) or muscle wasting
- Fatigue, weakness, functional decline
- Skin breakdown, recurrent infections

Assessment / Investigations

- Screening: Mini Nutritional Assessment (MNA)
- Weight, BMI, mid-arm circumference
- Labs: albumin, prealbumin (nonspecific but supportive)
- Assess for dysphagia, depression, dental issues

Management

Non-pharmacological:

- Individualized meal plans with preferred foods
- Nutrient-dense snacks between meals
- Oral nutritional supplements (e.g., high-calorie shakes)
- Feeding assistance and social dining programs
- Treat depression, pain, constipation that limit intake

Pharmacological:

1. **Appetite stimulants only if non-drug measures fail:**
   - Mirtazapine 7.5–15 mg HS (if insomnia/depression co-exist)
   - Megestrol acetate 160–320 mg/day (limited benefit; ↑ risk of DVT, edema)
2. Avoid routine use of stimulants due to side effects; focus on reversible factors first

References (Open-Access)

- NHS – Malnutrition: https://www.nhs.uk/conditions/malnutrition/
- Public Health Agency of Canada – Nutrition for Seniors: https://www.canada.ca/en/public-health
- Canadian Malnutrition Task Force: https://nutritioncareincanada.ca

CHAPTER 28
Constipation Management

Overview

Constipation is very common in LTC, affecting up to 50% of residents. It results from immobility, low fiber/fluid intake, medications, and comorbidities. Complications include fecal impaction, delirium, urinary retention, and bowel obstruction.

Risk Factors / Epidemiology

- Advanced age, immobility, dehydration
- Low fiber intake
- Medications: opioids, anticholinergics, calcium/iron supplements
- Neurological disease (Parkinson's, dementia, stroke)

Clinical Presentation

- Infrequent or difficult stools (<3/week)
- Hard, lumpy stools; straining
- Abdominal discomfort, bloating
- Overflow diarrhea in severe impaction

Assessment / Investigations

- History, medication review, bowel diary
- Abdominal and rectal exam (impaction)
- Rule out secondary causes (hypothyroidism, hypercalcemia)

Management

Non-pharmacological:

- Ensure hydration (≥1.5 L/day if not contraindicated)
- High-fiber diet (fruits, vegetables, whole grains)
- Encourage mobility/exercise if possible
- Toileting schedule after meals; privacy and comfort
- Address underlying pain, depression

Pharmacological:

- Bulk-forming agents: Psyllium 3.4 g PO daily (only if adequate fluids)
- Osmotic laxatives: Polyethylene glycol 17 g PO daily; Lactulose 15–30 mL PO daily–BID
- Stimulants: Senna 8.6–17.2 mg PO HS PRN; Bisacodyl 5–10 mg PO/PR daily–BID
- Suppositories/enemas for refractory constipation
- Opioid-induced: Naloxegol 25 mg PO daily; Methylnaltrexone 8–12 mg SC q48h

References (Open-Access)

- NHS – Constipation: https://www.nhs.uk/conditions/constipation/
- Public Health Agency of Canada – Seniors and bowel health: https://www.canada.ca/en/public-health
- Canadian Society of Intestinal Research: https://badgut.org

CHAPTER 29
Gastroesophageal Reflux Disease (GERD)

Overview

GERD is caused by reflux of gastric contents into the esophagus, leading to symptoms of heartburn, regurgitation, and complications such as esophagitis or strictures. In LTC, atypical presentations (cough, aspiration) are common.

Risk Factors / Epidemiology

- Obesity, hiatal hernia
- **Medications**: anticholinergics, calcium channel blockers, benzodiazepines
- Supine position after meals
- Older age with impaired esophageal motility

Clinical Presentation

- Heartburn, regurgitation, dyspepsia
- Chronic cough, hoarseness, aspiration risk
- Dysphagia, odynophagia if severe
- Complications: strictures, Barrett's esophagus

Assessment / Investigations

- Clinical diagnosis based on history
- Trial of PPI often diagnostic and therapeutic
- Endoscopy if alarm features (bleeding, weight loss, dysphagia, anemia)

Management

Non-pharmacological:

- Upright posture after meals (avoid lying flat for 2–3 hours)
- Elevate head of bed 15–30°
- Small, frequent meals; avoid late-night eating
- Avoid triggers: caffeine, alcohol, chocolate, fatty foods
- Weight management if obese

Pharmacological:

- Antacids PRN (aluminum hydroxide, calcium carbonate)
- H2 blockers: Ranitidine withdrawn; Famotidine 10–20 mg PO BID
- PPIs: Omeprazole 20 mg PO daily; Pantoprazole 40 mg PO daily; use lowest effective dose
- Long-term risks: fractures, C. difficile, hypomagnesemia; review need regularly

References (Open-Access)

- NHS – Acid reflux and GERD: https://www.nhs.uk/conditions/heartburn-and-acid-reflux/
- Public Health Agency of Canada – Digestive health: https://www.canada.ca/en/public-health
- Canadian Digestive Health Foundation: https://cdhf.ca

G.) MEDICAL CONDITIONS COMMON IN LTC – MUSCULOSKELETAL

CHAPTER 30
Falls Prevention & Frailty Assessment

Overview

Falls are a leading cause of morbidity and mortality in LTC residents. Frailty, defined as decreased physiologic reserve, increases fall risk and poor outcomes. Prevention strategies focus on multifactorial risk assessment and interventions.

Risk Factors / Epidemiology

- Age >80, frailty, sarcopenia
- Medications: sedatives, antipsychotics, antihypertensives
- Cognitive impairment, delirium, depression
- Impaired vision, neuropathy, arthritis, stroke, Parkinson's
- Environmental hazards (poor lighting, clutter, lack of grab bars)

Clinical Presentation

- Recurrent falls, near-falls
- Gait instability, dizziness, orthostatic hypotension
- Decline in ADLs, fear of falling

Assessment / Investigations

- Falls history (frequency, circumstances, injuries)
- Frailty scales: Clinical Frailty Scale (CFS), FRAIL questionnaire
- Gait/balance: Timed Up and Go (TUG) test
- Orthostatic BP, vision/hearing check, medication review

- Labs: vitamin D, CBC, electrolytes if unexplained falls

Management

Non-pharmacological:

- Exercise/physiotherapy (strength, balance, gait training)
- Vitamin D 800–1000 IU daily; calcium 1000–1200 mg/day
- Environmental modifications: grab bars, lighting, safe footwear
- Medication review and deprescribing high-risk drugs
- Staff education and fall prevention programs

Pharmacological:

- No specific drugs; review polypharmacy
- Treat underlying contributors (e.g., midodrine 2.5–5 mg PO TID for refractory orthostatic hypotension under specialist guidance)

References (Open-Access)

- NHS – Falls prevention: https://www.nhs.uk/conditions/falls/
- Public Health Agency of Canada – Falls in seniors: https://www.canada.ca/en/public-health/services/falls.html
- Canadian Frailty Network: https://www.cfn-nce.ca

CHAPTER 31
Hip Fracture Rehabilitation

Overview

Hip fractures are common in LTC and associated with high mortality and functional decline. Rehabilitation focuses on pain control, mobility restoration, and secondary fracture prevention.

Risk Factors / Epidemiology

- Advanced age, osteoporosis, female sex
- Frailty, dementia, Parkinson's disease
- Prior falls, poor vision, malnutrition
- Polypharmacy (sedatives, antihypertensives)

Clinical Presentation

- Acute hip pain after fall
- Inability to bear weight, shortened externally rotated leg
- Postoperative: pain, delirium, immobility, infections

Assessment / Investigations

- X-ray pelvis/hip to confirm fracture
- Pre/post-op labs: CBC, electrolytes, renal function
- Pain and mobility assessment
- Nutritional status evaluation

Management

Non-pharmacological:

- Early mobilization with physiotherapy (within 24–48h post-op)
- Multidisciplinary rehab (PT, OT, nursing, dietitian)

- Fall prevention strategies; hip protectors
- Nutrition: high protein diet, vitamin D and calcium supplementation

Pharmacological:

- Analgesia: Acetaminophen 500–1000 mg PO q6h PRN (max 3 g/day in elderly)
- Opioids (lowest dose, short term if severe pain): Morphine 2.5 mg PO q4h PRN; Hydromorphone 0.25–0.5 mg PO q4–6h PRN
- Avoid long-term opioids; add laxatives if used
- Thromboprophylaxis: Enoxaparin 30 mg SC daily or Dalteparin 5000 units SC daily (adjust for renal function)
- Osteoporosis treatment: Bisphosphonates or Denosumab if appropriate

References (Open-Access)

- NHS – Hip fracture: https://www.nhs.uk/conditions/hip-fracture/
- Osteoporosis Canada – Secondary fracture prevention: https://osteoporosis.ca
- Public Health Agency of Canada – Seniors and falls: https://www.canada.ca/en/public-health/services/falls.html

CHAPTER 32
Chronic Pain (Arthritis, Neuropathy)

Overview

Chronic pain in LTC is common due to arthritis, neuropathy, and musculoskeletal conditions. It reduces quality of life and mobility, and is often undertreated. Management balances efficacy with minimizing side effects.

Risk Factors / Epidemiology

- Osteoarthritis, rheumatoid arthritis
- Diabetes (peripheral neuropathy)
- Stroke, Parkinson's, post-herpetic neuralgia
- Falls and fractures, immobility

Clinical Presentation

- Persistent joint pain, stiffness, limited mobility
- Burning, tingling, numbness in neuropathic pain
- Depression, insomnia, functional decline due to pain

Assessment / Investigations

- Pain scales (Numeric, Visual Analog, PAINAD for dementia)
- Assess impact on ADLs, mood, sleep
- Review medications and contributing comorbidities

Management

Non-pharmacological:

- Physiotherapy, stretching, heat/cold therapy
- Mobility aids, supportive footwear

- Cognitive-behavioral therapy and relaxation techniques
- Occupational therapy for joint protection

Pharmacological:

- **Osteoarthritis:** Acetaminophen 500–1000 mg PO q6h PRN (max 3 g/day); topical NSAIDs (Diclofenac gel 1% applied QID)
- **Neuropathic pain:** Gabapentin 100–300 mg PO HS (renal adjust; max 900 mg/day in elderly); Duloxetine 30 mg PO daily (up to 60 mg)
- **Opioids:** Reserve for severe refractory pain; start very low (e.g., Morphine 2.5 mg PO q4h PRN)
- **Adjuvants:** Capsaicin cream topically; Amitriptyline 5–10 mg HS (limited by anticholinergic burden)

References (Open-Access)

- NHS – Arthritis: https://www.nhs.uk/conditions/arthritis/
- Canadian Pain Task Force – Chronic pain resources: https://www.canada.ca/en/health-canada/services/pain.html
- Public Health Agency of Canada – Seniors' pain management: https://www.canada.ca/en/public-health

CHAPTER 33
Mobility and Physiotherapy

Overview

Mobility support and physiotherapy are essential in LTC to preserve independence, prevent complications of immobility, and enhance quality of life. Programs should be individualized and multidisciplinary.

Risk Factors / Epidemiology

- Frailty, sarcopenia, arthritis
- Neurological disease (stroke, Parkinson's, dementia)
- Depression, social isolation
- Polypharmacy causing sedation or hypotension

Clinical Presentation

- Gait instability, difficulty with transfers
- Muscle weakness, contractures
- Falls, functional decline
- Pressure ulcers, venous stasis with immobility

Assessment / Investigations

- Functional assessment: Barthel Index, Katz ADL
- Gait/balance tests (TUG, Berg Balance)
- Physiotherapy assessment of strength, ROM
- Review mobility aids and environment safety

Management

Non-pharmacological:

- Physiotherapy: strength, balance, gait, transfer training
- Occupational therapy: adaptive devices, wheelchair seating
- Exercise programs (chair-based, resistance bands)
- Encourage mobility after meals and social activities
- Fall prevention integration

Pharmacological:

- Not directly applicable; optimize pain management and bone health (vitamin D, osteoporosis therapy) to facilitate mobility

References (Open-Access)

- NHS – Physiotherapy: https://www.nhs.uk/conditions/physiotherapy/
- Canadian Physiotherapy Association: https://physiotherapy.ca
- Public Health Agency of Canada – Physical activity for older adults: https://www.canada.ca/en/public-health

3. INFECTIOUS DISEASES IN LTC

CHAPTER 34
Influenza Prevention & Outbreaks

Overview

Influenza is a highly contagious respiratory illness with significant morbidity and mortality in LTC residents. Outbreaks can spread rapidly in communal living settings. Vaccination, early detection, and outbreak protocols are critical.

Risk Factors / Epidemiology

- Age >65, frailty, multimorbidity
- Immunosuppression, chronic lung/heart disease
- Close living quarters, unvaccinated staff/residents
- Seasonal outbreaks (fall/winter)

Clinical Presentation

- Sudden onset of fever, cough, sore throat, myalgia, fatigue
- Atypical in elderly: confusion, anorexia, functional decline

Assessment / Investigations

- Clinical diagnosis during outbreaks
- Nasopharyngeal swab for PCR/rapid antigen testing
- Monitor vitals, O2 saturation, hydration status

Management

Non-pharmacological:

- Isolate symptomatic residents; droplet/contact precautions
- Cohort staff; restrict visitors during outbreak
- Promote hand hygiene, masks, environmental cleaning

Pharmacological:

1. **Antivirals within 48h of symptom onset or for outbreak prophylaxis:**
   - Oseltamivir 75 mg PO BID × 5 days (treatment); 75 mg PO daily (prophylaxis)
   - Adjust dose if eGFR <60 mL/min
2. **Supportive care:** hydration, antipyretics (acetaminophen)

References (Open-Access)

- Public Health Agency of Canada – Influenza: https://www.canada.ca/en/public-health/services/diseases/flu-influenza.html
- NHS – Flu: https://www.nhs.uk/conditions/flu/

CHAPTER 35
COVID-19 in Nursing Homes

Overview

COVID-19 disproportionately affects LTC residents, with high mortality. Prevention relies on vaccination, infection control, and outbreak management. Treatment is supportive with antivirals and oxygen therapy as indicated.

Risk Factors / Epidemiology

- Advanced age, frailty, dementia
- Chronic diseases (lung, heart, kidney, diabetes)
- Immunosuppression
- High transmission risk in communal living

Clinical Presentation

- Fever, cough, dyspnea, anosmia, fatigue
- Elderly may present with delirium, anorexia, functional decline

Assessment / Investigations

- Nasopharyngeal PCR/antigen test
- Monitor O2 saturation; CXR if pneumonia suspected
- Labs: CBC, CRP, renal/hepatic function if severe

Management

Non-pharmacological:

- Isolation, PPE, cohorting of residents and staff
- Hand hygiene, visitor restrictions
- Encourage vaccination/boosters for residents and staff

Pharmacological:

- **Mild/moderate with risk factors:** Nirmatrelvir/ritonavir (Paxlovid) 300/100 mg PO BID × 5 days (avoid if severe renal/hepatic impairment; multiple drug interactions)
- **Severe disease (hospitalized):** Dexamethasone 6 mg PO/IV daily × up to 10 days
- **Oxygen:** Maintain SpO2 90–94%
- Avoid antibiotics unless bacterial co-infection suspected

References (Open-Access)

- Public Health Agency of Canada – COVID-19: https://www.canada.ca/en/public-health/services/diseases/coronavirus-disease-covid-19.html
- World Health Organization – COVID-19: https://www.who.int/emergencies/diseases/novel-coronavirus-2019

CHAPTER 36
Clostridioides difficile Infection (CDI)

Overview

Clostridioides difficile infection is a major cause of diarrhea in LTC, often linked to antibiotic or PPI use. It can cause severe colitis, dehydration, and recurrence. Prevention focuses on antibiotic stewardship and infection control.

Risk Factors / Epidemiology

- Recent antibiotic use (fluoroquinolones, clindamycin, cephalosporins)
- PPI use, immunosuppression
- Advanced age, comorbidities
- Outbreaks in LTC facilities

Clinical Presentation

- Watery diarrhea, abdominal pain, fever
- Leukocytosis, dehydration
- Severe cases: ileus, toxic megacolon, sepsis

Assessment / Investigations

- Stool test for C. difficile toxin/PCR
- CBC, electrolytes, creatinine
- Abdominal imaging if ileus or toxic megacolon suspected

Management

Non-pharmacological:

- Isolation, hand hygiene with soap/water (not alcohol-based)
- Environmental cleaning with sporicidal agents
- Stop inciting antibiotics if possible
- Hydration and electrolyte correction

Pharmacological:

- **First episode, non-severe:** Vancomycin 125 mg PO QID × 10 days OR Fidaxomicin 200 mg PO BID × 10 days
- **Severe:** Same as above; consider hospitalization
- **Recurrent:** Vancomycin taper/pulse regimen OR Fidaxomicin; fecal microbiota transplant in select cases

References (Open-Access)

- Public Health Agency of Canada – C. difficile: https://www.canada.ca/en/public-health/services/diseases/clostridium-difficile.html
- CDC – C. difficile: https://www.cdc.gov/cdiff

CHAPTER 37
Skin/Soft Tissue Infections

Overview

Skin and soft tissue infections (SSTIs) are common in LTC, often related to pressure injuries, poor hygiene, or chronic edema. They range from cellulitis to abscesses and can lead to sepsis in frail elderly.

Risk Factors / Epidemiology

- Diabetes, peripheral vascular disease
- Chronic wounds, pressure ulcers
- Poor hygiene, incontinence, edema
- Immunosuppression, malnutrition

Clinical Presentation

- Local erythema, warmth, swelling, tenderness
- Fever, leukocytosis in systemic infection
- Abscess: fluctuant, purulent drainage
- Necrotizing infection: severe pain, rapid progression, systemic toxicity

Assessment / Investigations

- Clinical diagnosis
- Wound swabs if purulent drainage
- Blood cultures if systemic signs
- Imaging (US/CT) if abscess or necrotizing fasciitis suspected

Management

Non-pharmacological:

- Wound care and debridement if necessary
- Pressure ulcer prevention strategies
- Elevation of affected limb, compression for edema
- Infection control precautions in facility

Pharmacological:

- Mild cellulitis: Cephalexin 500 mg PO QID × 5–7 days
- Severe/systemic: Ceftriaxone 1 g IV daily; Vancomycin IV if MRSA risk
- Abscess: incision and drainage; add antibiotics if systemic signs
- Necrotizing fasciitis: emergency transfer; broad-spectrum IV antibiotics

References (Open-Access)

- NHS–Cellulitis: https://www.nhs.uk/conditions/cellulitis/
- Public Health Agency of Canada – Wound and skin infections: https://www.canada.ca/en/public-health
- CDC – Skin infections: https://www.cdc.gov/mrsa

CHAPTER 38
Vaccination Protocols (Influenza, Pneumococcal, Shingles, COVID-19)

Overview

Vaccination is essential in LTC to prevent outbreaks and protect vulnerable residents. Routine immunization reduces morbidity, hospitalizations, and mortality.

Recommended Vaccines

- **Influenza:** Annual vaccination for all residents and staff
- **Pneumococcal:** PCV20 or sequential PCV15 + PPSV23 as per national guidelines
- **COVID-19:** Primary series and boosters as recommended by public health
- **Shingles (Herpes zoster):** Recombinant zoster vaccine (Shingrix) 2 doses, 2–6 months apart
- **Tetanus/diphtheria/pertussis (Tdap): Booster** every 10 years if not up-to-date

Implementation in LTC

- Facility-wide vaccination campaigns
- Staff education and consent process for residents
- Documentation and monitoring of vaccine uptake
- Outbreak protocols and rapid vaccination when recommended

References (Open–Access)

- Public Health Agency of Canada – Vaccination: https://www.canada.ca/en/public-health/services/vaccination.html
- NHS – Vaccinations for older adults: https://www.nhs.uk/conditions/vaccinations/
- CDC – Vaccines and immunization: https://www.cdc.gov/vaccines

4. SKIN / WOUND CARE

CHAPTER 39
Pressure Ulcer Prevention and Treatment

Overview

Pressure ulcers (pressure injuries) are localized damage to skin and underlying tissue due to prolonged pressure, shear, or friction. They are common in immobile LTC residents and associated with pain, infection, and mortality.

Risk Factors / Epidemiology

- Immobility, frailty, advanced age
- Malnutrition, dehydration, incontinence
- Diabetes, vascular disease
- Poor positioning or inadequate pressure relief surfaces

Clinical Presentation

- Redness or non-blanchable erythema (Stage 1)
- Blister/partial thickness skin loss (Stage 2)
- Full-thickness skin loss with subcutaneous involvement (Stage 3)
- Exposure of bone/muscle (Stage 4)
- Pain, odor, drainage; possible cellulitis or osteomyelitis

Assessment / Investigations

- Regular skin checks (Braden Scale for risk)
- Wound assessment: size, depth, exudate, infection signs
- Swab/culture if infection suspected
- Imaging if osteomyelitis suspected

Management

Non-pharmacological:

- Repositioning every 2 hours; off-loading devices (pillows, foam wedges)
- Pressure-relieving mattresses/cushions
- Optimize nutrition (protein, vitamins, hydration)
- Moist wound healing with appropriate dressings (hydrocolloid, foam, alginate)
- Debridement of necrotic tissue (surgical, enzymatic, autolytic)

Pharmacological:

- Analgesia: Acetaminophen 500–1000 mg q6h PRN (max 3 g/day in elderly)
- Topical antimicrobials for infected wounds (silver dressings)
- Systemic antibiotics only if cellulitis, sepsis, or osteomyelitis

References (Open-Access)

- NHS – Pressure ulcers: https://www.nhs.uk/conditions/pressure-sores/
- Public Health Agency of Canada – Seniors and skin health: https://www.canada.ca/en/public-health
- Canadian Association of Wound Care: https://www.woundscanada.ca

CHAPTER 40
Diabetic Foot Care

Overview

Diabetic foot complications result from neuropathy, ischemia, and infection, leading to ulcers and amputations. Prevention and early management are crucial in LTC to preserve mobility and quality of life.

Risk Factors / Epidemiology

- Diabetes with poor glycemic control
- Peripheral neuropathy, peripheral arterial disease
- Poor footwear, foot deformities
- Prior ulcers or amputations

Clinical Presentation

- Numbness, tingling, pain, or loss of protective sensation
- Ulcers (often plantar surface), calluses, infections
- Poor wound healing, gangrene in severe ischemia

Assessment / Investigations

- Daily foot inspection by staff/residents
- Monofilament or tuning fork for neuropathy
- Pulses, capillary refill; ABI if PAD suspected
- Swab if ulcer infected; X-ray for osteomyelitis if deep

Management

Non-pharmacological:

- Daily inspection, hygiene, moisturizing (avoid between toes)
- Proper footwear and off-loading of pressure areas
- Regular podiatry care; nail trimming
- Education of staff and residents

Pharmacological:

- Optimize glycemic control (avoid hypoglycemia)
- Antibiotics for infected ulcers: Cephalexin 500 mg PO QID × 7–10 days; or Clindamycin 300 mg PO TID (if penicillin allergy)
- Severe infections: IV antibiotics (ceftriaxone, vancomycin if MRSA risk)
- Topical antimicrobials not routinely recommended unless mild superficial infection

References (Open-Access)

- NHS – Diabetic foot problems: https://www.nhs.uk/conditions/diabetic-foot-problems/
- Public Health Agency of Canada – Diabetes and foot care: https://www.canada.ca/en/public-health
- Diabetes Canada – Foot care resources: https://www.diabetes.ca

CHAPTER 41
Common Skin Cancers

Overview

Skin cancers, particularly basal cell carcinoma (BCC), squamous cell carcinoma (SCC), and melanoma, are common in elderly LTC residents. Early detection and referral are essential.

Risk Factors / Epidemiology

- Age, fair skin, chronic sun exposure
- Immunosuppression, prior skin cancer
- Genetic predisposition

Clinical Presentation

- BCC: pearly papule, telangiectasia, central ulceration
- SCC: scaly erythematous plaque or nodule, ulcerated lesion
- Melanoma: asymmetric, irregular border, color variation, >6 mm, evolving lesion (ABCDE criteria)

Assessment / Investigations

- Full skin exam during routine care
- Dermoscopy if available
- Biopsy for suspicious lesions
- Staging for melanoma if invasive

Management

Non-pharmacological:

- Sun protection (hats, clothing, sunscreen)
- Staff education to recognize suspicious lesions

- Regular skin checks in LTC

Pharmacological/Surgical:

- Referral for excision/dermatology
- BCC/SCC: surgical excision or cryotherapy
- Melanoma: wide excision; oncology referral for advanced cases
- Topical 5-fluorouracil or imiquimod for superficial BCC/SCC in select cases

References (Open-Access)

- NHS – Skin cancer: https://www.nhs.uk/conditions/skin-cancer/
- Canadian Cancer Society – Skin cancer: https://cancer.ca
- Public Health Agency of Canada – Sun safety: https://www.canada.ca/en/public-health

CHAPTER 42
Pruritus & Xerosis

Overview

Pruritus (itching) and xerosis (dry skin) are frequent in LTC, often due to aging skin, dehydration, or systemic disease. Though usually benign, they can significantly impair quality of life and cause skin breakdown.

Risk Factors / Epidemiology

- Advanced age, low humidity, dehydration
- Diabetes, CKD, liver disease, thyroid disease
- Medications: opioids, diuretics
- Poor skin care or hygiene practices

Clinical Presentation

- Generalized or localized itching
- Dry, flaky, cracked skin (xerosis)
- Excoriations, lichenification from scratching
- Secondary infections (cellulitis, impetigo)

Assessment / Investigations

- History, review of medications
- Physical exam for xerosis, dermatitis, infection
- Labs: CBC, renal/liver/thyroid function if systemic cause suspected

Management

Non-pharmacological:

- Regular emollients (fragrance-free creams/ointments)
- Short, lukewarm showers; avoid harsh soaps
- Humidifiers in dry environments
- Gentle clothing and bedding

Pharmacological:

- Topical corticosteroids for dermatitis (Hydrocortisone 1% cream BID × 1–2 weeks)
- Oral antihistamines for itch interfering with sleep: Cetirizine 5–10 mg PO daily or Hydroxyzine 10–25 mg PO HS (sedating)
- Treat systemic cause if identified (optimize renal/hepatic/thyroid function)
- Antibiotics for secondary infection if needed

References (Open-Access)

- NHS – Itchy skin (pruritus): https://www.nhs.uk/conditions/itchy-skin/
- Canadian Dermatology Association – Dry skin and itch: https://dermatology.ca
- Public Health Agency of Canada – Seniors and skin health: https://www.canada.ca/en/public-health

5. MENTAL HEALTH & SOCIAL ISSUES IN LTC

CHAPTER 43
Social Isolation and Loneliness

Overview

Social isolation and loneliness are highly prevalent among LTC residents and are linked to depression, cognitive decline, and increased mortality. COVID-19 exacerbated these issues due to visitor restrictions. Addressing social needs is as important as medical care in LTC.

Risk Factors / Epidemiology

- Widowhood, lack of family support
- Cognitive impairment, dementia, depression
- Sensory impairments (vision, hearing loss)
- Mobility limitations, immobility
- Language/cultural barriers

Clinical Presentation

- Withdrawal from activities
- Depressed mood, apathy
- Poor appetite, sleep disturbances
- Decline in functional and cognitive status

Assessment / Investigations

- Geriatric Depression Scale, UCLA Loneliness Scale
- Social history, support networks
- Assess barriers: hearing, vision, mobility

Management

Non-pharmacological:

- Encourage group activities, recreational therapy
- Volunteer visits, pet therapy, music therapy
- Technology support for video calls with family
- Address sensory deficits with glasses, hearing aids

Pharmacological:

- No specific drugs; treat underlying depression/anxiety if present
- Antidepressants: SSRIs (e.g., Sertraline 25–50 mg PO daily) if indicated

References (Open-Access)

- NHS – Loneliness in older people:
  https://www.nhs.uk/conditions/loneliness-in-older-people/
- Public Health Agency of Canada – Social isolation and seniors:
  https://www.canada.ca/en/public-health/services/health-promotion/aging-seniors.html

CHAPTER 44
Elder Abuse & Neglect

Overview

Elder abuse includes physical, emotional, financial, sexual abuse, or neglect. It is underreported in LTC and has devastating consequences. Healthcare workers are mandatory reporters in most jurisdictions.

Risk Factors / Epidemiology

- Cognitive impairment, dementia
- Dependence on caregivers
- Social isolation
- Caregiver stress, burnout, lack of training

Clinical Presentation

- Unexplained bruises, fractures, burns
- Fearfulness, withdrawal, depression
- Poor hygiene, malnutrition, pressure ulcers
- Financial exploitation (sudden money changes)

Assessment / Investigations

- Careful history; interview resident alone if possible
- Physical exam for injuries
- Documentation with photos if permitted
- Involve social work and legal authorities as required

Management

Non-pharmacological:

- Ensure immediate safety of the resident
- Report suspected abuse to appropriate authorities

- Provide psychosocial support and counseling
- Staff training on elder rights and respectful care

Pharmacological:

- Not applicable except treating injuries or associated depression/anxiety

References (Open-Access)

- World Health Organization – Elder abuse: https://www.who.int/news-room/fact-sheets/detail/elder-abuse
- Government of Canada – Elder abuse: https://www.canada.ca/en/public-health/services/health-promotion/aging-seniors/elder-abuse.html

CHAPTER 45
Family Involvement in Care

Overview

Family involvement in LTC improves resident well-being, satisfaction, and quality of care. Collaboration between staff and families supports person-centered care and advance care planning.

Risk Factors / Epidemiology

- Families may experience guilt, stress, or conflict with staff
- Lack of communication can reduce involvement
- Cultural differences influence expectations

Clinical Presentation

- Residents benefit from advocacy, emotional support
- Families may notice changes earlier than staff
- Lack of involvement may lead to poorer outcomes

Assessment / Investigations

- Family meetings, care conferences
- Review care goals and advance directives
- Assess caregiver stress

Management

Non-pharmacological:

- Regular communication and updates
- Involve families in ADLs and decision-making
- Education on disease processes and prognosis
- Encourage participation in recreational activities

- Support caregiver mental health

Pharmacological:

- Not applicable; focus on psychosocial support

References (Open-Access)

- NHS – Social care and support guide: https://www.nhs.uk/conditions/social-care-and-support-guide/
- Government of Canada – Supporting caregivers: https://www.canada.ca/en/public-health/services/caregivers.html

CHAPTER 46
Culturally Sensitive Care

Overview

Culturally sensitive care recognizes residents' diverse backgrounds, beliefs, and values. It fosters dignity, trust, and inclusivity in LTC facilities.

Risk Factors / Epidemiology

- Increasing diversity among LTC residents
- Language barriers, health literacy gaps
- Cultural differences in care expectations and decision-making

Clinical Presentation

- Miscommunication, mistrust of healthcare providers
- Non-adherence to treatment plans due to cultural beliefs
- Stress in families when cultural needs are unmet

Assessment / Investigations

- Cultural assessment during admission (language, diet, spiritual needs)
- Involvement of interpreters and cultural liaisons
- Review care goals in culturally sensitive framework

Management

Non-pharmacological:

- Respect dietary restrictions, religious observances
- Provide interpreter services when needed

- Staff cultural competence training
- Incorporate cultural practices into care plans
- Engage community resources and spiritual leaders

Pharmacological:

- Not directly applicable; adapt medication discussions to health literacy and beliefs

References (Open-Access)

- World Health Organization – Cultural competence in health care: https://www.who.int
- Government of Canada – Culturally appropriate health care: https://www.canada.ca/en/public-health

6. PRACTICAL NURSING CARE IN LTC

CHAPTER 47
Medication Safety in LTC

Overview

Medication errors are common in LTC due to polypharmacy, frailty, and cognitive impairment. Ensuring medication safety involves accurate prescribing, dispensing, administration, and monitoring, with a focus on deprescribing where appropriate.

Risk Factors / Epidemiology

- Polypharmacy (>5 drugs)
- Cognitive impairment, communication barriers
- High-risk drugs: anticoagulants, insulin, opioids, sedatives
- Transitions of care, poor documentation

Clinical Presentation

- Adverse drug events: falls, delirium, bleeding, hypoglycemia
- Medication non-adherence
- Functional decline, hospitalizations

Assessment / Investigations

- Medication reconciliation at admission and transitions
- Regular medication reviews with physician/pharmacist
- Use tools: Beers Criteria, STOPP/START
- Monitor labs (renal/hepatic function, INR, glucose)

Management

Non-pharmacological:

- Staff education on safe medication administration
- Clear labelling and secure storage of meds
- Avoid pill splitting/crushing unless safe
- Double-check high-alert medications (insulin, warfarin)
- Encourage deprescribing of unnecessary drugs

Pharmacological:

- Adjust doses for renal/hepatic function
- Simplify regimens (once daily where possible)
- Use blister packs or automated dispensing systems

References (Open-Access)

- Canadian Deprescribing Network:
  https://deprescribing.org
- NHS – Medicines safety:
  https://www.nhs.uk/medicines/

CHAPTER 48
Monitoring Vitals & Early Warning Signs

Overview

Regular monitoring of vital signs helps detect early deterioration in LTC residents. Early warning scores can support timely interventions and reduce hospital transfers.

Risk Factors / Epidemiology

- Frailty, multimorbidity
- High risk of sepsis, pneumonia, heart failure
- Cognitive impairment masking symptoms
- Medication side effects

Clinical Presentation

- Subtle changes: confusion, decreased mobility, anorexia
- Vital sign abnormalities: fever, tachycardia, tachypnea, hypoxemia, hypotension
- Early signs of infection, heart failure, dehydration

Assessment / Investigations

- Routine monitoring: BP, HR, RR, O2 sat, temp, pain scale
- Early Warning Systems (NEWS2) adapted for LTC
- Nursing documentation of trends
- Rapid response for acute deterioration

Management

Non-pharmacological:

- Train staff to recognize early deterioration
- Escalation protocols for abnormal vitals
- Regular hydration/nutrition checks
- Family communication when deterioration detected

Pharmacological:

- Treat underlying cause: antibiotics for infection, diuretics for CHF, fluids for dehydration
- Avoid unnecessary hospital transfers when palliative approach preferred

References (Open-Access)

- NHS – National Early Warning Score (NEWS2): https://www.rcplondon.ac.uk/projects/outputs/national-early-warning-score-news-2
- Public Health Agency of Canada – Seniors' health: https://www.canada.ca/en/public-health

CHAPTER 49
Pain Assessment in Non-Verbal Patients

Overview

Pain is under-recognized in LTC residents with dementia or communication barriers. Validated observational tools are essential for assessment to ensure adequate pain relief.

Risk Factors / Epidemiology

- Dementia, aphasia, severe illness
- Frailty, immobility, pressure ulcers, fractures
- Post-surgical states

Clinical Presentation

- Facial grimacing, guarding, withdrawal
- Agitation, aggression, restlessness
- Changes in sleep, appetite, mobility

Assessment / Investigations

- Tools: PAINAD (Pain Assessment in Advanced Dementia), Abbey Pain Scale
- Regular nursing observations during care
- Rule out infection, constipation, fractures as pain causes

Management

Non-pharmacological:

- Positioning, pressure relief
- Heat/cold packs, massage, physiotherapy
- Distraction: music, activity

Pharmacological:

- Stepwise approach: Acetaminophen 500–1000 mg PO q6h PRN (max 3 g/day)
- NSAIDs rarely used; risk of GI bleed, renal dysfunction
- Opioids: Morphine 2.5 mg PO q4h PRN; Hydromorphone 0.25–0.5 mg PO q4–6h PRN (short term)
- Adjuvants: Gabapentin 100 mg HS (neuropathic pain); Duloxetine 30 mg daily if tolerated

References (Open-Access)

- NHS – Pain management: https://www.nhs.uk/conditions/pain/
- Canadian Pain Task Force: https://www.canada.ca/en/health-canada/services/pain.html

CHAPTER 50
Infection Prevention & Control

Overview

Infection control is critical in LTC to protect vulnerable residents from outbreaks. Standard precautions, vaccination, and antimicrobial stewardship are central components.

Risk Factors / Epidemiology

- Frailty, advanced age, immunosuppression
- Close living quarters, shared equipment
- Indwelling devices (catheters, feeding tubes)
- Poor hand hygiene or environmental cleaning

Clinical Presentation

- Increased infection risk: pneumonia, UTIs, gastroenteritis, C. difficile
- Outbreaks: influenza, COVID-19, norovirus

Assessment / Investigations

- Routine surveillance of infections
- Staff screening during outbreaks
- Audit hand hygiene and cleaning protocols

Management

Non-pharmacological:

- Hand hygiene with soap/alcohol rubs
- PPE during outbreaks
- Isolation/cohorting of symptomatic residents
- Environmental cleaning and disinfection

- Education and training for staff

Pharmacological:

- Antimicrobial stewardship: avoid unnecessary antibiotics
- Vaccinations: influenza, pneumococcal, shingles, COVID-19

References (Open-Access)

- Public Health Agency of Canada – Infection prevention and control:
  https://www.canada.ca/en/public-health/services/infectious-diseases.html
- CDC – Infection control in LTC:
  https://www.cdc.gov/longtermcare

CHAPTER 51
Documentation in LTC

Overview

Accurate documentation is essential in LTC for continuity of care, legal protection, and quality improvement. Records must be clear, factual, timely, and compliant with standards.

Best Practices

- Document care promptly after delivery
- Use objective, factual language
- Include resident's condition, interventions, and response
- Record vitals, medications, ADLs, incidents
- Avoid jargon, ensure legibility in handwritten notes

Electronic Documentation

- Increasing use of EMRs in LTC
- Ensure accuracy, confidentiality, and compliance with privacy laws
- Use structured templates and checklists

Legal and Ethical Considerations

- Documentation is a legal record
- Omissions may imply care was not provided
- Residents have the right to access their records
- Maintain confidentiality (HIPAA, PHIPA compliance)

References (Open-Access)

- NHS – Record keeping and documentation: https://www.nhs.uk/common-health-questions/nhs-services-and-treatments/how-to-access-your-medical-records/
- Government of Canada – Health information privacy: https://www.canada.ca/en/health-canada/services/health-concerns/health-privacy.html

www.ingramcontent.com/pod-product-compliance
Lightning Source LLC
Chambersburg PA
CBHW040927210326
41597CB00030B/5209